NUTRITION *IN A* NUTSHELL

This book is dedicated to my gorgeous friends Mark and Charlotte. You are beautiful people in every single way! Thank you for always shining with positivity and smiles and being there to support me in everything I do.

First Printing: August 2015

ISBN: 978-1-326-51645-1

Tough Cookie Publishing

Email: info@toughcookieblog.co.uk

www.toughcookieblog.co.uk

Ordering Information:
Special discounts are available on quantity purchases by corporations, associations, educators, and others. For details, please contact the publisher at the above listed address.

U.S. trade bookstores and wholesalers: Please contact Tough Cookie Publishing at the above listed address.

CONTENTS

I. About Me

I had an incredibly negative relationship with myself for over a decade until I decided that I had to start trying to change things around for myself. I had Anorexia when I was 14, and whilst I recovered fully from that I was never able to shake off the demons which forced me to believe I wasn't good enough - to hate myself and the way I looked. Ever since my recovery I have wanted to help others by offering a positive, honest perspective on the world – and a huge part of what I do is helping all women (and men!) to feel better in their own skin in a world which increasingly encourages us to scrutinise and 'improve' ourselves.

Although there were lots of different triggers behind me developing Anorexia, one of the biggest things I struggled with at the time even before I was poorly was the fact that I felt horrendously fat, coupled with awful diet advice I found in magazines and newspapers which gave me a warped perception of how I 'should eat'. Vulnerable and susceptible, how could I have known anything different? We had weren't educated about nutrition at school, and so I spent hours poring over these articles which advised me to eat cereal for lunch and soup for dinner. What drives me to talk about the way I eat now and food in a positive light is the fact that these articles still exist – diet companies still exist – and while they exist in the way that they do currently, I'm sure many people will continue to have a distorted view of how they 'should look' and how they 'should eat' – as I did for years before I discovered the truth.

What I'm really passionate about is stopping eating disorders before they begin; and whilst as I say there are many factors which cause people to develop Anorexia I think a good knowledge of food and nutrition is a good place to start for all of us when we decide we want to have a healthier relationship with our bodies – whether we've been through an eating disorder or not.

Tough Cookie was created to help anyone to feel better about themselves, but specifically to offer inspiration and support to those suffering with Anorexia. Through Tough Cookie I aim to challenge the stereotype of what is 'normal' and 'beautiful' and prove that it is possible to live a full, happy and healthy life - even if you've not always had the best relationship with your body and mind.

2. About this book

I believe that changing your perspective on food and your body can change your life.

This book isn't a diet book. It's not a scientific, medical view of our bodies and what we put in them either. It's about sharing my perspective to help others – a perspective which has taken me a long time to develop, but which has been shaped by my experiences with food and my relationship with it over the years.

Imagine how it would be if you didn't feel you needed to 'watch your weight'? Imagine never going on a diet ever again (and never wanting to!) Imagine being able to understand your body better and enjoy your food without wondering what's in it or whether it will make you 'fat'. Knowing that your body is healthy and nourished and feeling happy from the inside out. Not feeling the need to control and limit and ban and cut out.

I wrote this book along with my other book, Tough Love, to help people to achieve that state of 'letting go' of the vice grip we have on our bodies and on food – forcing ourselves to eat in a certain way because we are misguidedly following a set of ridiculous rules. I wrote the books because I know how it feels to be controlled by an obsession with food and a belief that I wasn't 'beautiful' or 'good enough' – that I was fat and ugly. Now I know the truth about myself and about food – and so can you! Understanding nutrition and learning about your body is the best place to start.

Why did I write this book?

For those who don't know me or don't know my books and the blog, bringing out a nutrition book and recipe books seems crazy when they hear that just a few years ago, food was most definitely not my friend – let alone an ally and collaborator which not only saw me discover physical strength I never knew I had, but also helped me to achieve my lifelong dream of publishing books and helping other people to feel better about themselves.

At the age of 14 and consumed by Anorexia, I was convinced that I would never have a healthy relationship with food. I think myself so lucky to be here and to have discovered a love for food as I have, but I think being so close to death actually brings you closer to life – in addition to giving you the gift of a unique perspective on a range of things, which of course includes nutrition and body image in particular. But this perspective didn't develop overnight following my recovery – it took years.

Ever since my experience with Anorexia I have wanted to help others in the same situation. What I'm also passionate about is improving each and every person's relationship with their body and with food – a relationship which I believe has deteriorated in the age of the rat race, saturated with diets, processed and convenience foods, and a society consumed by the media's perception of how we all should look and what size we should be.

Why is nutrition so important to me?

As an Anorexic 14 year old I was understandably struggling with the concept of food and how to eat. Yet as a 17 year old college student, a 19 year old make-up artist and a 21 year old writer, I'd still have told you that a cup soup for lunch and a bag of Haribo for dinner was the way forward. Now I'm incredibly passionate about nutrition – having learnt so much more about the body and how anything less than a nourishing, balanced lifestyle isn't fair or healthy mentally or physically.

What I eat is really important to me now – for all the right reasons! Around 8 years after my recovery and still confused about food and its role in my body (and my life), I developed a keen interest in nutrition. I believe that a good understanding of how our bodies work and what we eat is really important for everyone – not just people who are vulnerable or who are recovering from an eating disorder.

Back then I was eating a very poor diet and regularly went without eating enough, skipping meals and constantly buying branded diet foods because I was afraid of becoming fat. Even though I was staying the same weight and wasn't poorly, I wasn't healthy either. Then four years ago, I developed Irritable Bowel Syndrome. I started reading about the effect eating the way I did was having on my whole body. Now I have a better understanding of nutrition and how my body works I'm really interested in the physical consequences of our obsession with image as well as the psychological, and I want to share how I look after my body and why because of the various health issues I've had over the years to help other people in similar positions.

In addition to promoting positivity and recovery from Anorexia, I wanted to educate myself and others on the power of nutrition and advocate a healthy relationship with food – especially for young people who are vulnerable and often influenced by the crap we're fed by the media and diet companies.

We only get one body - and after what I've been through I'm more conscious of that than ever. In honesty, I think owing to the stressful lifestyles we all live, not many people quite feel their best – and that is partly down to how we eat and our relationship with food.

I'm learning how to live with myself, mentally and physically – and nutrition is such an important part of that journey.

Why is this book different?

This book is not about losing weight, keeping fit or cutting things out. It's different because it's been written by someone who had Anorexia and battled with a negative personal outlook for years – with food being a large part of that. This book is different because it touches on the link between self-esteem, society and food, and has been written with better overall wellbeing in mind rather than just a singular physical or mental change. After discovering more about my body and my mind how they are so delicately linked, now I appreciate food and nutrition and want to look after myself. I researched a lot over the years to develop the view I hold now of nutrition, and spent time making sure that this book is as balanced and positive as possible.

Often we take our health for granted, but really it's the most precious thing we have. We only realise how essential optimum health is for our daily function when it is taken away from us – even in an insignificant way. Whether it's something as small as a cold, a water infection or even a hangover, feeling under the weather even slightly can affect us massively. Good nutrition can aid our health immensely – without the right balance of nutrients, our bodies aren't best placed to fight illness, deal with the day-to-day or be the best they can be physically or mentally in order for us to live our lives to the full. Whilst you might think dieting, starvation, excessive exercise and looking like a VS model is what 'healthy' is all about, hopefully with this book I'll show you a different perspective.

For those who have had Anorexia

If you're reading this book after having had Anorexia or Bulimia, your body has just been through something incomprehensible, and it will need to be rebuilt slowly and with lots of care and attention.

Until 2 years ago, I still knew nothing at all about nutrition. I recovered with no medical help – I wasn't on a refeeding plan and I wasn't monitored. Once I decided I wanted to get better, I began eating as much as I could, of the unhealthiest foods I could get my hands on, in an effort to put weight back on. I was fixated on the number on the scale and counting calories: in the opposite way. Only now do I know how dangerous that was – and that I should have been monitored closely and refed carefully until I was out of danger.

I say in Tough Cookie that weight means nothing, but when you are recovering from Anorexia, weight becomes everything. That's partly the measure of how healthy you are becoming. But there's more to becoming healthy again than simply putting on weight – I believe it's about feeding your body with the best possible nutrients to help you get back on your feet again and repair any damage done.

I perish the thought of stuffing my face with so many processed refined foods when my body was dying and needed the best quality food I could give it.

Over the past few years I've been asked by members of my family, friends and acquaintances how and why I eat like I do. I always promote a healthy relationship with food which doesn't involve cutting things out, weighing food, counting fat or calories (or counting anything, for that matter) and which is centred around eating natural, wholesome foods which provide some sort of nourishing benefit for the body. I believe that if you concentrate on the quality of food and not quantity, the body looks after itself. I don't believe in starvation, I don't eat anything I don't like – good nutrition should be for life, it shouldn't be temporary. It shouldn't be about chewing on raw veg miserably and skipping meals to achieve a short-term goal only to binge on sweets when you've reached that goal. I'm not here to say you can't eat this or don't eat that – then I'd be just as bad as a diet company myself. This book promotes the concept of balance and sensible eating, all with a goal of a better relationship with food. Hopefully here you'll also find the tools to help you to achieve and understand that rather than being fearful of it.

So what about everyone reading this who doesn't have or has never had an eating disorder?

If you haven't suffered from an eating disorder, maybe you're reading this book because you're fed up with feeling bad about yourself and confused over your diet, and want to eat simple, tasty, wholesome food without feeling guilty. Perhaps you just want to learn more about nutrition. That's the best thing though: this book isn't just for those recovering from eating disorders – it's for everyone who wants to help their bodies to be the best they possibly can be and to be as healthy as they can be, inside and out.

When I talk to women (and a lot of men) I often hear that they are on a 'diet'. Something which they believe is a healthy lifestyle change (albeit commonly with a questionable motive of weight loss behind it). They tell me proudly how they've skipped breakfast today or had a diet yoghurt for lunch - and then I have to explain the horrified look on my face! I want to change that. Seeing people struggle miserably following these ridiculous regimes, crippled with low energy levels munching down on something which they think is good for them but is actually doing more harm than good upsets me. Knowing what I know now and seeing all this crap 'advice' makes me so angry. When I talk to people who think they're making the right choices and are desperately trying to be healthy, I really feel it is incredibly unfair that they should be misinformed in this way and compromise their health unknowingly when they think they're doing the right thing. My goal is to challenge the misinformation circulated by diet companies and encourage everyone to live happily, healthily and at peace with their bodies as much as is possible – without focusing on weight.

What worries me possibly more than this is that we are inadvertently teaching our next generations to be obsessed with weight and unhappy with their bodies - as shocking statistics showed recently that over 60% of school-age girls had been on a diet or felt 'fat'.

So what can we do about this? Aside from promoting positive self-esteem (that's what my other book Tough Love is about) I think a good knowledge of basic nutrition is needed in order for anyone to understand their bodies better and learn how harmful modern day diets with the motive of weight loss behind them can be. It's a slightly unconventional perspective to be introduced to after being exposed for so long to a common way of thinking about food – I understand that. But hopefully everything in this book makes sense and enables you to ignore the adverts for diets, dismiss the irresponsible magazine articles and instead live life to the full. A healthy relationship with food is the first step to a healthy lifestyle – and that's what the diet industry *won't* tell you.

3. What is nutrition, why is it so important, and how could it change your life?

What is nutrition?

Nutrition is simply defined as 'the process for providing food necessary for health and growth'. More academically-speaking it's the practice and study of how food benefits us, and how our bodies work in relation to what we eat.

I believe that nutrition has been over-complicated by the media and diet companies over the years. A lot of the things people *think* they know about food and the way they eat are actually untrue – but when that's what they've been told for years and years, who can blame them? I'm still learning every day about how my body works but now, being more educated than I ever was, I shudder when I think of how I used to eat even after I'd recovered from Anorexia; skipping meals, living off sweets and fizzy diet drinks in an effort to stay slim. I was still reading the shit in magazines about 'being healthy' – spending huge amounts of money on branded diet foods believing one hundred percent that they were good for me because they kept me 'thin'.

A society obsessed with image and wanting to lose weight is a breeding ground for fad diets and a general ignorance when it comes to good nutrition. I understand that it's easy to be pulled in and tempted by a quick fix, especially when under pressure to look 'perfect' - I've been there. But the phrase 'too good to be true' is never more relevant than when it comes to commercial diets. The best way really is eating healthily, keeping active and concentrating on the *quality* of the food you eat not the quantity – that's all there is to it. There's more hard work involved, but in the long run what's more appealing?

Nutrition does not mean dieting and good nutrition shouldn't be difficult, complicated or detrimental to your health. 'Diets' are upsetting to me, because healthy eating shouldn't be temporary or harmful in any way. And by 'healthy eating' I don't mean starvation or living off salad. Your body is your most important asset – without it you're pretty stuck. You live in it day in, day out; yet few of us respect it or take into consideration the hundreds of thousands of processes that take place every second just to keep us alive. Our bodies do this without us even having to do a single thing consciously or physically – we don't even have to think about it. Most of us are completely unaware of at least half the processes that are going on continuously to keep us functioning properly. Our only responsibility really (apart from avoiding vices such as smoking and general danger) is eating properly and drinking enough. Let's face it – how many of us get that right?

We don't get it right because we're simply not educated on how to get it right. We can be forgiven for our ignorance, because we are not biologists, doctors or nutritionists. If we were, the diet industry certainly wouldn't be as big as it is – in fact it'd probably be non-existent. How can we possibly be expected to go against everything we have ever been taught about food?

Whether you are liberated from society's ideals and the diet industry's view of food or not, we're still told that food and nutrition is confusing and complex – a science which is only employed by medical professionals and body builders.

Nutrition however doesn't need to be complicated at all. Eat fresh, natural, whole foods, don't over- or under-eat and indulge in a treat now and again. Feed your body when it asks for food and try to make sure that you're eating something worth eating – giving your body what it is asking for, what it needs – energy, vital nutrients and minerals. That's all pretty simple – but the *difficult* bit is getting your head around that and at the same time ignoring the incorrect information you've learnt over time – but that's where this book comes in.

It's impossible to underestimate the effects of diet on every element of your whole body (and your life) – from hormones and brain function, to energy levels and the maintenance of healthy hair and skin.

Why is nutrition important – and why do we know so little about it?

Food becomes an enemy when you have Anorexia - it is an inconvenience to say the very least – a road block to your destination. I found myself not only enraged with my body, but with food itself, with meals, with modern culture and with anybody who ate normally or encouraged me to do the same. Yet for everyone, no matter what their health complaint, mental or physical, nutrition is important. Many modern illnesses and health phenomenon are now being attributed to our poor diets and (sometimes unintentional) abuse of our bodies.

It's important to establish firstly that food is not the enemy. It's actually your best friend – and it constitutes a large part of your role in taking care of your body. It should simply be seen as something needed to sustain your life, fuel for your body, but also something to be enjoyed. Maybe you think you'll never see it that way now, but there are, however, things that you can do to improve your relationship with food.

To say it is difficult maintaining a healthy relationship with food in today's society would be an understatement. That's why nutrition is so important. The messages that we are given about how to think about food and the role it plays in our lives are mostly negative and revolves around how food makes us look aesthetically, not how it makes us *feel* or how it nourishes us biologically-speaking. Most 'health conscious' press and advice we are exposed to is a thinly-veiled attack on food, whether that's a certain type or group of food, the way we eat, or the time we eat. We're constantly told how to eat, what to eat and when to eat.

This constant scrutiny of our diets and the way in which we eat makes us crave control over it. We feel bad if we do not have control over our diets. This leads to obsession, on a society wide scale, not just on a personal level.

Really, we shouldn't think extensively about food at all. As cavemen and women, our only thoughts on food were where our next meal would come from. Tribes in remote corners of the earth often survive on a diet that many of us would find unpalatable for a variety of reasons. But their focus is purely on survival; and nothing else.

The damage of the diets and heavily-processed foods that have plagued society since the 40s and 50s has done extensive damage to the way we eat and the way we think about eating. For many, food is a bit of a pain and an inconvenience.

What I believe in is eating well to nourish your body – eating good, wholesome food which provides your body with much needed energy and nutrients which allow you to live a happy, healthy life. I've learnt that if you concentrate on the quality of your food and not the quantity or the numbers, your body will take care of itself. You will look and feel good. You'll see later on in 'Diets and The Fall Out with Food', that the way you eat should be for life; it shouldn't be temporary. The focus should be on your health and happiness, not on the way you look. If you look after these important elements, that will come naturally. Choosing wholesome, natural food and seeing how it benefits your body will make a huge difference to you.

I can honestly say that out of all the products and topical treatments I've tried for skin, hair and nails, nothing beats a good diet. I can't express the negative effects of my diet over the years on my appearance; after all, being 'thin' really isn't all there is to a person on the inside OR on the outside. You might already know that with being underweight comes pale, sallow skin, thinning hair, digestive problems, and that's just for starters. Being overweight involves increased risk of heart attack, diabetes, lymph issues and joint issues. If that's what's apparent on the outside, then you can only imagine what sort of damage has been done on the inside. Eating well, eating often and eating enough has always made rapid improvements to my overall health and appearance.

It's for this reason that I am now passionate about nutrition and eating well. It's changed my perspective on food massively because I found that when I managed to let go and not count calories and fat and only look at the origin of my food and try to choose natural things, I didn't suddenly become 'fat' or 'ugly' or gain weight. I just had more energy and felt freer, at liberty to choose and eat what I wanted. That's why nutrition is important – because it can have a positive effect on your whole life – not just on the way you feel or how you look.

How could understanding nutrition and developing a better relationship with food change your life?

Before I learned about nutrition, I was trapped in a cycle of eating poorly, then wondering why my skin was dry, my hair fell out and I lacked any energy. I was so frightened of putting on any weight that I weighed myself once a week and sometimes if I was heavier I tried to lose half a stone if I felt particularly 'big'. I never thought about food as nutrition or as something which could benefit me in any way – instead, I thought of it as numbers. I thought of it as 'good' and 'bad'. I rarely ate breakfast and even though I worked 12 hour days on my feet I'd sometimes go all day with only a cereal bar to sustain me. At the time, I thought it felt good. Being slim was good, feeling hungry was good, lacking energy was good. But when I look back now, I can see that really it was all bad. I wasn't living my life because I was so tired all the time, and I was miserable because I was constantly hungry.

Eventually I got a job which involved me sitting down a lot – and I struggled. I worried I'd gain weight and now I was in an office environment, so I was tempted to snack to pass the time. I started going to the gym and loved the tough classes but I realised I was hungrier – I'd need to eat more if I wanted to train hard. Then I started to struggle with certain foods when I increased my intake. I found I couldn't eat much more without having terrible stomach pain and I wasn't able to go to the toilet. After a few trips to the GP I was diagnosed with Irritable Bowel Syndrome. It was anxiety related, and as I have Generalised Anxiety Disorder which was worse at the time, I found myself bloated and in pain constantly. I started to worry about eating because I knew I'd feel poorly – so I picked at stuff and ate my way around the foods I wouldn't have touched before. I'd regularly just eat the cream out of cream-cakes and buy loads of sweets just to get me through the afternoon. I tried lots of different diets and supplements and went to my GP for medication several times – but nothing worked.

It was only when I started reading online about IBS that I realised how distorted my view of food was. Naturally a lot of the articles discussed good nutrition from a more factual, medical perspective, and soon I was reading blogs and studies on websites which explained how the human body works and how different foods are processed. I started to understand that years of liquid dieting, starvation and sugar binges could have made the issues I had now inevitable. I knew for sure that I had been so wrong to treat my body so badly.

It took a little while for me to let go of the anxiety around not controlling my food and ditching the diet and processed stuff in favour of everything full fat, raw and natural – things without labels on or calories attached. But this (and a better understanding of my relationship with myself) changed my life dramatically.

For the first time since my eating disorder I didn't experience hair loss of any kind. My skin glowed. I had more energy. I actually felt stronger and developed a real passion for food. I created recipes for all the things I loved but couldn't eat anymore because of my IBS and they were ten times more nutritious than the cakes and cereal bars I'd lived off before. Most of all, my body didn't change like I'd been worried it would – even when I stopped going to the gym so much.

Having even a basic appreciation of nutrition and how wrong the information we all consume on a daily basis is had a huge impact on my quality of life – and liking myself better physically helped me to improve my mental wellbeing, too.

I ask you at the beginning of the book to imagine not being worried about food. Think about how it would be to eat without panicking, to never feel like you're starving yourself, to be full of energy and full of life. Knowing your body and yourself better allows you to just that – without worrying that you are being unhealthy or getting fat.

Nutrition and self-esteem

One of the reasons why I am particularly passionate about nutrition is that I feel it is intrinsically linked with our self-esteem. Because diet companies and years of negative media have affected our relationship with food and our bodies, perhaps irreversibly, most people see 'food' as something negative to be controlled and limited in order to look good.

Most people I know have been or are on some sort of diet – and when I ask why, they all have similar motives. *'Oh, I just want to be a little slimmer', 'I just want to lose a few pounds', 'I'd like to be more toned'.* They're completely unaware that whatever their goals may be, they are misguided – and what's more, they aren't seeing themselves as they really are – men and women alike.

Nutrition and self-esteem go hand in hand – and when you improve one, you automatically improve the other. Which you tackle first of course depends entirely on you as we are all different – but they must both be the best they can be if you want to live your life to the full. I really hope that you read this book and it helps you to feel better and shed some positive, truthful light on food and the diet industry. However if you are still struggling and feel you need support with your self-esteem to stop dieting or to feel better about the way you look, then please head over to my blog for inspiration and take a look my book Tough Love, in which share my experiences to help anyone with low self-esteem and body dysmorphia to live their lives to the full.

4. Please don't diet

Diet companies and the fallout with food

The fallout with food

Food, for many of us, has become an inconvenience. For most, no longer does it mean a lovingly prepared meal that is placed on the table in the evening, or a therapeutic afternoon spent baking with the kids. Instead it is a frantic stabbing of a fork into plastic, the furious jabbing of the well-worn numbers on a microwave at 8 o' clock in the evening, skipped breakfasts, crippling indigestion and the hoarding of low-fat yoghurts and diet cereal bars reserved for when we have the energy to 'diet'.

Having had an eating disorder, you see food from a completely new perspective. Now I see with clarity a culture which soured my relationship with food and led me to go to a dangerous extreme using food as a bomb with which to self-destruct. I was so frustrated and angered by food – I saw it as something which made me fat and disliked. I followed the frankly irresponsible and largely contradictory advice offered up by glossy magazines in the hope that I would look like the celebrities which I longed to emulate, in order to be approved of by others. As adults and as children, our perception of food is simply as fat and calories and as good and bad, and we are not actually aware of how it is really used in our bodies and how important a good diet is for us to function properly.

Food is so important for me now. Not only have I always loved cooking and baking, I also find it fascinating how we fit food into our lives with some irritability yet it has such a huge effect on us in so many ways. What we eat is often a last-minute thought or a hastily made decision based on tenuous information – despite the fact that our bodies are our most vital asset – the only place we have to live in. They're the most important thing we can spend our time and money on – as without your health, what can you do and who can you be? Nutrition is still hugely misunderstood and even government guidelines on what we should be eating tend to be vague and generalised and don't actually inform us of how beneficial eating the right foods can be to our mental and physical wellbeing.

After I clued up on nutrition and began to develop wholesome recipes to replace the things I could no longer eat, I started to share them with my friends and family. They couldn't believe that they could possibly come under the bracket of 'healthy' – even less so when I explained the ingredients contained within them, and why they were nutritious.

I think that's because generally people's perception of what is healthy is skewed to think that anything 'low fat' or 'low calorie' is good for us when in fact, the opposite is true. Wholefoods, such as nuts, vegetables, meat, and unprocessed dairy all contain a wealth of nutritious goodies - vitamins and minerals which enable all of our bodily functions to work as best they possibly can. Because they are usually eaten as nature intended, they often contain a perfect balance of nutrients. I don't count calories or fat anymore – I don't even look on the back of packets. Generally I don't have to – the food I buy is in its raw state and sometimes doesn't even come in packets! For someone who has had an eating disorder and who lived in a world of disordered eating and packet-reading, it's a huge departure – and one which I hope I share with you in this book to inspire you to see food differently, in a positive light.

What we eat (and enjoying what we eat) has such a huge effect on our mental health as well as how we feel and look. For example, did you know that peanuts and oats can help to increase serotonin production (as anti-depressants do)? Or that pure cocoa powder contains more antioxidants than fruit juice?

I'm not saying for a second that food is any substitute for medication. But just rekindling the joy of food and realising what it means for our overall health for me is a huge step for anybody – not just those who are in recovery from an eating disorder or any other serious mental or physical health condition.

Weight is just a number

The first things to cover before we dive into the harmfulness of dieting is the focus of diets: weight, and size. Weight is now very much an indicator for health, the 'measuring stick' for most diet regimes, which inevitably means it's become an obsessive focus for many women who continually weigh themselves, never happy with the number on the scale.

There are a few reasons why the 'weight' mentality is all-wrong.

Firstly from a medical perspective, the number on the scale is not an accurate indication of overall health. A weight can only tell us a limited number of things about the body. A full analysis of our health would involve a number of tests, including a check of body fat levels using instruments and callipers, blood tests, measurements taken from vital areas such as the waist and then a resulting calculation. 'Weight loss' is never a healthy perspective to come from. It implies that it doesn't matter what you're losing, as long as the number on the scales decreases.

You could chop off a limb and lose a lot of weight – but it's fairly likely you wouldn't be pleased about that! It's an extreme example, but it demonstrates that the number on the scale will go up and down and will be affected by a number of factors – some you can see, some you can't. For women especially hormonal changes and water retention can alter the result. The weight of our bodies depends on many different factors and varies from hour to hour, day to day, week to week. Don't forget the contribution of our digestive systems to how much (or little) we weigh. We should actually focus on good health – and nothing else. When you realise that your whole worth and beauty is not based upon that, you will be much healthier mentally and physically.

If your goal is toning up and reducing in size, the only accurate way to understand your progress at the gym is to have a professional use fat callipers or other technology which will give you a clear picture of how much fat you have in relation to muscle, and where it is on your body, so that you can train smarter not harder.

When you focus solely on weight, you're not focusing on health, nutrition, muscle tone or metabolism, simply the number on a scale, which never gives us an accurate or positive reflection of ourselves mentally or physically. Yes, BMI is calculated from weight – but what that and your magic number don't tell you is what's going on *inside* your body. For example going on weight and BMI alone, a body builder could be classed as obese. That's because if he is short in height, but carries a lot of muscle (which is dense and pound for pound 'heavier' than fat), he may weigh more than a person who is the same height, but has little muscle and a lot of fat. If you went off their weights alone, you'd probably say the second man was healthier – but in actual fact it's the first. So you see, weight really is a vague indicator when it comes to overall health and fitness.

An example of why focusing only on weight can actually result in a less healthy individual, it's worth noting that fitter people tend to weigh more than people of the same size and build without any muscle mass. If you want to tone up, chances are you may end up weighing more. Many people are disheartened when after weeks of eating right and hard gym sessions they're seeing the number on the scale creeping up. However this is common – it is a good sign and can mean that your body is building muscle. As before, you can be heavier, but slimmer – because weight doesn't show what you're made of inside.

Before I stopped weighing and measuring myself obsessively, I noticed that after joining the gym I gained 10lbs. My measurements were exactly the same, if not a little smaller. But I felt physically better than I ever had done before – mentally too. Laying store by a number on a scale does nobody any good. How many diets focus on how you feel and what you have to gain? Not many? How many instead focus on what you have to lose? Lose 3lbs, 5lbs, 10lbs in 2 weeks. The unfortunate truth is, you may stand to lose a lot more than pounds.

Weight, plainly speaking, is simply your relationship with gravity. Of course, it means so much more than that for most of us. For many people (myself included until just a year or so ago), the number on the scale means the difference between being happy with how we look, and being unhappy with how we look. Just a few pounds either side of your 'ideal number' can make a huge difference to your mood and your self-esteem. I don't weigh myself anymore – but before I stopped, I lost count of the times I gained a pound and felt fat and miserable for the rest of the day – or lost a pound and felt like a supermodel for a few hours. We seem to be shackled by this harmful obsession with weight, so much so that it seems to be all many people talk about and a huge focus in their lives.

Weight is essentially just a number. It doesn't tell you anything else other than what you actually physically weigh in relation to other objects on the earth. More importantly, it doesn't reflect or reveal anything about you as a person. It doesn't take into account any other physical or personal qualities. A number on a scale won't reveal how wonderful you are. It won't show your kindness, humility, your sense of humour. We're placing a lot of value by something that really doesn't equate to that much of ourselves.

Weighing and measuring causes us to compare. Whilst it's not something I'll cover in this book, in Tough Love I talk about comparison a lot, and how it's almost never a fair thing to do to yourself, as you'll always look at yourself unfavourably in relation to others. Weighing yourself religiously can also de-motivate you. If you're constantly weighing yourself and don't see results (or see a gain or loss when you were hoping for the opposite), a poor result can actually cause a drop in morale. It often causes you to indulge in bad habits – like not eating enough or eating the wrong types of food in order to get that number lower. These habits not only harm our metabolism and other bodily functions, but they also hamper your mission for good health.

The bottom line is: You could be doing more harm than good if you only focus on the number on the scale.

Diets and weight

Diets and weight are intrinsically linked – and their symbiotic relationship is one which often results in people feeling miserable and becoming trapped in a series of everlasting diets.

Diets always focus on your current weight, and how much you have to lose. They set (often unrealistic) goals which can result in misplaced happiness or shame depending on whether they're reached or not.

Often the weight loss which is expected of people who enrol in diet schemes is totally unreasonable. They're given an irresponsible representation of what they weigh now and what they 'should' weigh – irrespective of any other external or internal factors which may affect that. Healthy people are often bullied into feeling as though they 'need' to lose one, two, three stone – when in fact they're perfectly healthy as they are. So they embark on a fad diet and lose the weight far too quickly – only to find that they then can't come off the diet as they need to continue eating abnormally just to maintain their current weight. Inevitably this type of thing makes participants miserable and self-conscious, but it also makes it likely they'll gain and store more fat in the long run.

With group-based diets weight loss also becomes a competition. Although the advertised 'benefits' of these groups are that you are supported by other members, in actual fact everyone is competing with each other and using other people's failures to feel better about themselves – and there's nothing healthy about that.

Sizing

Although this hasn't strictly got anything to do with nutrition, I do think sizing has a small place in this book. It's something I discuss in more detail in Tough Love, because often people define themselves by their size and use it as a 'measuring stick' for weight loss. The problem with this is that sizes differ depending on the shop and type of clothing you're buying.

Anyone who has ever been clothes shopping will know that it's not uncommon to be a size 10 in one shop, and a size 14 in another. This was something which always used to bother me – because in my head, sizes were grouped into 'fat' and 'thin.' A 'thin' size would be anything between a 4 and a 10, and a 'fat size' was 12 and above. I was a size 12-16, so in my head I was 'fat'. This was ridiculous obviously, but that's the impression I'd been given from magazines, celebrities and skinny friends.

The other issue with sizing is that one person can be several different sizes even in just one shop, or for one item of clothing. This depends on how we're built – as women especially some of us have bigger chests, or very thin legs. I use myself as an example for this because my own size difference is pretty extreme. I have a 24 inch waist – but I also have 37 inch hips. This means that I am a size 6-8 (XS-S) on top, and a 12-16 (L – XL) on the bottom – cue shopping nightmares. But I don't feel bad about having to buy XL or Size 16 for my bottom half, because I understand now that I am not a 'fat' size, that's just the way I am built.

Disordered eating and bad habits

After dieting or an eating disorder you'll naturally have a distorted idea of food – but what many people don't realise is that they have a warped perception of diet and nutrition even though they've never been on a proper 'diet' or suffered from Anorexia or Bulimia.

Have you ever skipped breakfast consistently hoping to lose weight? Eaten cereal or taken liquid supplements twice a day to drop a jeans size? Cut out certain foods for fear of them making you 'fat'? That's disordered eating.

Disordered eating is defined as an abnormal relationship with food, albeit in a relatively less dangerous way than an eating disorder. It's anything that deviates from what would be classed as a 'normal' way of eating, for example, not really thinking about what you eat and when, eating a balance of foods in the right quantities. Despite the 'safer' status, disordered eating can cause long-term damage to your health. You might have guessed that some of the above examples are practices advocated by popular diets and celebrity gurus – hence my reasoning for the chapters which follow.

Often even when we stop a diet or don't go 'full blown' with one, we retain or develop associated bad habits. It becomes 'fashionable' or 'popular' to do a certain thing based on the advice being promoted at the time – so often whole groups of men and women find themselves being swept along, damaging their bodies as a result. Diets undoubtedly are behind widespread disordered eating, poorer health and self-esteem issues in the Western world – and that's why they always have a prominent place in my books.

Why I disagree with diets – and why they are bad for you

Diet shakes, soup diets, juicing, fasting – amongst my friends and family, my hatred of diets and diet foods is well known.

I talk earlier in this chapter about disordered eating. Most people wouldn't count themselves as having an eating disorder. Yet how many do you know have disordered eating? Do they ever skip breakfast deliberately to save calories? Have they ever done a liquid diet or eaten cereal twice a day instead of balanced meals? It's not an eating disorder of course; but it's not a normal, healthy relationship with food. How many of us who are a healthy weight are constantly watching what we eat in the hope of losing weight or for fear of putting it on? How many are encouraged to check the back of packets constantly, to check the calories, fat and carb content of their meal?

We are rightly told that eating disorders have a devastating effect on the human body. It's not as widely researched, publicised and documented, however, that eating abnormally over a long period of time (a lifetime, for some) can be detrimental in lots of ways for our health. Many people I know are on a constant diet - so what harm is this doing to their bodies? Moreover, what harm is this doing to their *minds*? Our bodies are not designed to live with temporary solutions, lurching from one strict discipline to the next. Generally when people diet, because it is a temporary 'solution' to a problem (supposedly your weight - 'diets' have one sole purpose and goal – to lose weight), they finish the diet and return to their old habits, expecting to retain the results. They are so relieved that this period of what is usually fasting and eating food they hate is over that the way they used to eat is amplified. So they put weight back on, and go back on another diet – probably a different type of weight loss. The cycle begins again. Think about what this does to our bodies – a vicious circle which is initiated by our thoughts about food.

It's also worth noting that despite the obsession many of us hold with food and how we look, obesity continues to be a concerning problem which is becoming a growing burden in the westernised world. I genuinely believe part of this is down to the same issues which I discuss here in the book – over-dependence on poor advice, processed food and a fixation on weight and diet which studies have shown actually causes people to end up fatter, not slimmer.

Diet is a dirty word

I really believe that diets and the diet industry as a whole has a lot to answer for when it comes to rising numbers of eating disorders, disordered eating and body dysmorphia and whilst it's a controversial and bold step to repeat this time and again in my books, I feel it's essential because it still shocks me when I talk to people (with or without eating disorders) how many of them believe what we are all told about our bodies and how they work – not to mention the aesthetic pressure and poor body image that diets promote.

I really dislike the word 'diet' because instantly, it has negative connotations. What is the first thing that pops into your mind when someone says diet? Hunger, eating vegetables, being miserable in order to 'look good'. They go against common sense; they encourage you to be unkind and damaging to your body in order to achieve a short term goal.

I'd go as far to say that pretty much every woman (and man) I meet is on a 'diet' of some sort. Desperately trying to lose weight, obsessed with food, poring over magazines, choking on dry brown toast at breakfast and downing a radio-active coloured smoothie at lunch because that's what they have been told to do - and at the end of that they see themselves posing on a beach in a bikini smiling just like the celebrities who feature in these magazines. But it comes at the expense of their happiness and ultimately, their health. This is because they take guidance from much-peddled nonsense about how we should 'lose weight' and in turn 'be healthy'. I see these as different beasts entirely.

Some people are morbidly obese. Clinically, they need to get below a certain weight and this is when the number on the scale matters. This is when strict portion control and the reduction of fats matter.

However, those who are a healthy weight take this advice on board to achieve their own goals; not realising that in actual fact treating your body in this way causes more harm than good in a relatively healthy person.

Yes, some diets are effective in helping people who need to lose weight, in the short-term at least. But at what cost? Rarely is the weight loss sustainable; as human beings can't live properly in a malnourished state for very long. Yo-yo dieting is on the increase because of this, a vicious cycle of losing the weight, putting it on, losing it again. This can lead to various long-term illnesses, digestive problems and hormonal imbalances. The emphasis is all wrong – and there is no focus in any media on being fit, strong and healthy.

Diet companies, as with the beauty companies and advertisers, make money by identifying something 'wrong' with you (in this case, they make you feel like anybody who isn't perfectly slender is 'wrong') which needs fixing. They offer products and services which will 'fix' this so-called 'defective' or 'undesirable' part of you. This is destructive to say the least. As you are more and more exposed to these images of who and how you should be, you become more and more desperate. You want a quick fix. The diet companies know this, so they fabricate a 'fast and easy' formula for you to follow which guarantees 'weight loss'. Have you noticed that they never mention health? Energy? Metabolism? Hormones?

Given my dim view of 'diets' in general, you can imagine that ones such as this which come with unpleasant side-effects and potentially harmful consequences are really not in favour with me. But what are the consequences of trusting regimes like this?

With liquid-based and starvation diets (naming no names), what you're losing rapidly is water, not fat. Your body also loses muscle tone and clings on to fat stores for dear life. In addition, the meal

40

replacements tend to be full of sugar and chemical nasties which are far from good for you.

With restrictive diets which force you to 'cut out' a whole food group (for example, carbs) the same applies – as your body is depleted of nutrients. It's also true of the diets which have you weighing everything out until you can't eat without knowing how many grams your meal is. With diets that encourage you to substitute real food for processed cereal filled with sugar. What all of these diets also have in common is they trap you. You lose the weight initially – mostly phantom, some 'real' (of course, because your body is effectively being starved), and then you get to a point where you have to 'come off' the diet and eat normally again. So when you do, your relieved body starts to become healthier again, replenishing the lost nutrients, hanging on to any fat and generally feeling confused.

The diets which perhaps cause the most lasting mental damage for each and every one of us are the diets that encourage you to count calories, or equally as harmful, points – branding certain foods as 'sinful' or 'harmful'. This forces us to put a false value on food and to become obsessed over counting the points or calories accordingly. We start to see meals as a value or as positive or negative and not as food – focusing on quantity over the quality. These diets promote and consequently develop such an unhealthy relationship with food, a belief system which once established is very difficult to break free from.

The way these diets operate makes them open to abuse. When you see food as quantity, you will 'save' your points, calories or whatever you are counting for foodstuffs which may not be the best for you, (a week of salads and dry toast in exchange for those 2 bottles of wine you're going to drink on Friday night, for example), with the mistaken belief that this is 'okay' because after all, that's what these diets preach. As long as you're coming in below a certain number each day, who cares what you're eating?

Losing weight using any method like this is really damaging for your body and overall health – that's without the horrific consequences that anyone who has had an eating disorder will appreciate well. What's more, it can cause irreparable damage to your metabolism and other important bodily functions and essential processes, including your digestive and reproductive systems.

It's very difficult coming back into the 'real world' recovering from an eating disorder (or changing your perspective after a lifetime of dieting) when it is full of this bullshit. It's hard not to obsess over food and crave control over our size, shape and weight when not only do diet companies and media ignore the possibility that what they promote can be harmful to mental and physical health, can cause body dysmorphia and other mental damage and can be a catalyst for eating disorders, they actively encourage it. But it can be done – I'm living proof of that.

In an ideal world I'd love to see more responsible practice and marketing where diets are concerned which take into consideration not just people who are vulnerable and prone to develop eating disorders and other issues, but *all* men and women. That day is unlikely to come, so it is down to us to see the world for what it really is – and media outlets who misinform us and diet companies for what they really are – businesses which make lots of money out of what is largely unhealthy misery.

My parting shot on diets is a question for everybody who hasn't had Anorexia or Bulimia. Would you trash your own house? Of course you wouldn't – you have to live in it every day. With diets, so many people wreck their bodies, often unintentionally – but unlike a house, we can't move out of our bodies. We only get one for life – so why would we be so irresponsible with it and make it a difficult place for us to live in?

Why diet food is bad for you

Do you know that you could be eating junk food without even knowing it? Consuming foods which won't benefit your body when you're consciously trying to do the opposite?

We're constantly told that certain foods are 'good for us' – 'low fat', 'no added sugar', 'gluten free', 'dairy free' but in fact much of this is a myth. Labelling is very clever – and just because it says 'natural' on the packet, it's unfortunately likely that your perception of natural and its actual definition in the food manufacturing world are poles apart. 'Natural', 'low-fat' and 'sugar free' have come to mean 'good for you' – so it's difficult to believe that they could mean the opposite.

One of my biggest issues with diet foods is that they encourage you to ditch healthy, natural nourishing alternatives with nothing wrong with them, swapping them for 'low fat' options which are actually bad for you. A small low-fat yoghurt, for instance, is filled with chemicals and sugar (sometimes as much as a chocolate bar), whereas full fat Greek yoghurt is packed with protein, good fats, vitamins and probiotics.

Gluten free and dairy free alternatives are also often highly processed and contain more chemicals and sugar than their 'original' counterparts – so unless you are intolerant, they're really not a savvy choice. Ironically, supermarkets charge a premium for these foods – so not only are you hurting your body, you're also hurting your finances too. There's more on this a little bit later in the book in Mythbusters.

What's the alternative?

Although it's rarely what people want to hear (human nature and impatient society dictate that we naturally favour a 'quick fix', with an 'all or nothing' mentality taking precedence over 'balance'), the only alternative to dieting and spending years miserably yo-yoing between 'good' and 'bad' weights is to challenge the thoughts and beliefs you currently hold about food so that you can eat without feeling fearful or wanting to control it.

For me, the first step to regaining a positive relationship with food and with your body is to learn more about it and try to see the things you've believed for years from a fresh perspective – and that's where this book comes in.

5. Nutrition – in a nutshell

I strongly believe that it might have been possible for me not to have developed an eating disorder if I had been exposed to some sound nutrition advice from a qualified nutritionist while I was at school. We never had access to anything like this; instead most of my (incorrect) information came from magazine articles and diet companies. As a consequence my idea of how my body worked and how it used food was warped beyond belief. We did cover food in biology and in citizenship but it was a vague, 'curriculum's-eye' view of nutrition and not something I could take anything practical away from. Being obsessed with food, I used to collect articles and avidly watch food programmes and read diet magazines because they added 'evidence' to my distorted opinion of food.

In this chapter I cover food in a very basic way and offer a no-bullshit idea of how food works in our bodies. I hope that being better informed makes a positive difference to how you think and feel about yourself. It might even inspire you to go on and learn more about your body and nutrition, as I did.

We've been taught a lot of myths about diet and nutrition, which have shaped the way we eat and think about food.

At its most basic, good nutrition involves each meal or snack you eat containing a good balance of food groups. A lot of natural foods tend to cover all three all on their own; nuts, for example, have a good measure of protein, fat and carbohydrate in them.

It's so simple – yet it's become invariably complicated for all of us.

Why does eating healthily feel difficult?

Partly the complication and confusion comes about because we live in the first world, in which we are lucky enough to have experienced lots of advances in the manufacture of foodstuffs over the years. Only 50 years ago many people didn't have fridges or freezers in which to store food – so it had to be bought and freshly prepared each day. Developments in our roles in modern life as women (and as men) have meant we simply don't have time to do that anymore. Convenience food has become king. Fresh, natural food is harder to come by – and has an appropriately high price tag to reflect this.

Every type of food which was once lovingly prepared from scratch with fresh natural ingredients now comes ready made in a packet with a long list of unrecognisable ingredients on the back of it. With ready meals, confectionery and anything else you can think of often containing a questionable balance of what our bodies need, as a society we are getting bigger and less healthy – and coupled with inactivity through increased time spent at desks and in front of televisions this leads to a health crisis. Unfortunately we have developed a terrible way of coping with that. We are inadvertently limiting the intake of the foods we need replacing them with processed alternatives, and as a consequence we're missing out on their benefits. We are becoming *less* healthy as a result, not *more* healthy. Obesity is on the rise, eating disorders are on the rise, poor self-esteem is rife and diabetes, heart disease and certain cancers are more prevalent than ever before. We don't understand that healthy means having a balance of everything we need; not a tiny waistline. As I say before – the emphasis is on 'weight', not good health; and as long as food fits the description of what we *think* is healthy (low fat, low carb, diet) then we understandably think that it must be good for us. Ironically, the absolute opposite is true.

What does eating healthily involve?

Before you can eat healthily, you need to understand what constitutes 'healthy'. I've already covered what's *not* healthy – dieting, skipping meals, starving yourself and eating diet foods. But what's the opposite of that? For lots of people, the words 'healthy eating' conjure images of munching raw broccoli and downing foul juices. But actually eating healthily should be fun. It should make you feel good inside and out. It shouldn't involve eating things which taste bad or make you feel poorly.

For me eating healthily involves challenging your current approach (eating more, eating better, loosening the need for control around food) and making healthy swaps most of the time. That means that you can in theory eat whatever you want – you can have anything in moderation. But reserve the foods which don't nourish your body (sweets, fast food, processed meals and salty snacks) for 'cheat days' or weekends – as long as the majority of what you eat is beneficial, it doesn't matter.

If you're looking for someone to tell you that it's 'easy' to lose weight, then you're reading the wrong book – that's not what this book is about! I'm not going to tell you there's such a thing as a 'quick fix' or a magical formula for being healthy (whatever that means to you), because they don't exist. You might think that they do – but actually these are schemes which underpromise and overdeliver, harming your body and your mental wellbeing in the process.

One thing which did help me to stop starving my body of nutrients without feeling frightened and as though I was making a massive change all at once was swapping.

Often swaps can seem like 'poor relations' or involve impractical or unconventional substitutes, so I've included a table of some of mine below to give you examples. In my recipe books I included the recipes I still make regularly – especially the cakes and desserts, because I didn't want to feel deprived.

Healthy Swaps

Swap: Diet chocolate biscuits

For: Healthy, easy to make home-made cookies

Why? Diet chocolate biscuits are likely to be just as bad for you as their 'full fat' alternatives - plus they'll be high in salt and preservatives. Home-made cookies are always better for you – but a healthy recipe allows you to enjoy them knowing you're benefitting nutritionally.

Swap: Crisps

For: Unsalted nuts

Why? It's no secret that crisps can be high in fat and salt. Unsalted nuts are high in healthy fats and contain plenty of protein and fibre.

Swap: Chips

For: Baked sweet potato fries

Why? Processed chips can contain trans-fats and high amounts of salt – you can make home-made versions with white or sweet potato using rapeseed oil, which retains its nutritional values at high temperatures.

Swap: Cake

For: Healthy, simple mug-cake

Why? Ready-made cakes are baked in factories in the same way biscuits are – so they will contain preservatives to keep them fresh plus high levels of refined sugar and salt. Making your own is easy and inexpensive and a healthy recipe guarantees nutritional benefit without the feeling of 'missing out.'

Swap: Ready Meals

For: Quick, simple easy meals which can be made in advance

Why? Ready meals are also made with lower quality ingredients, often with higher quantities of salt and sugar compared with meals you make yourself. If you're short on time make one-pot meals in advance and freeze them or try some quick, easy-to-prepare meal ideas for a change.

These are just conventional examples, but of course it depends on what you eat now and how you could do things differently. Perhaps you always find yourself snacking on cereal bars and fruit but want a healthier alternative without going hungry. It may be that you eat very well generally but never have time to cook so depend on ready meals – so the switch there would be to plan in advance and make and freeze your favourites.

A healthy balance

If you hear doctors or nutritionists speaking about diet, you'll often hear the word 'balance' included in their dialogue. That's because biologically the only way to look after your body is to adopt a measured approach to what you eat. That's difficult to hear if you're used to avoiding a certain food group, or genuinely believe that 'carbs are bad' or everything you eat should be 'non-fat'. But imagine if you lived solely on crisps, or bacon, or apples. You wouldn't be giving your body a balanced mix of the nutrients and vitamins it needs to function properly – and your digestive system wouldn't thank you, either. Although your limitations and restrictions may feel less extreme than the examples given above, they may be doing a similar type of damage to your body, and certainly aren't sufficiently nourishing you – your diet will definitely be lacking in something. I know I used to hate seeing the diagram below because it made nutrition seem complex, confusing and uncertain – and I felt it left me with nothing to control in order to make sure I stayed slim.

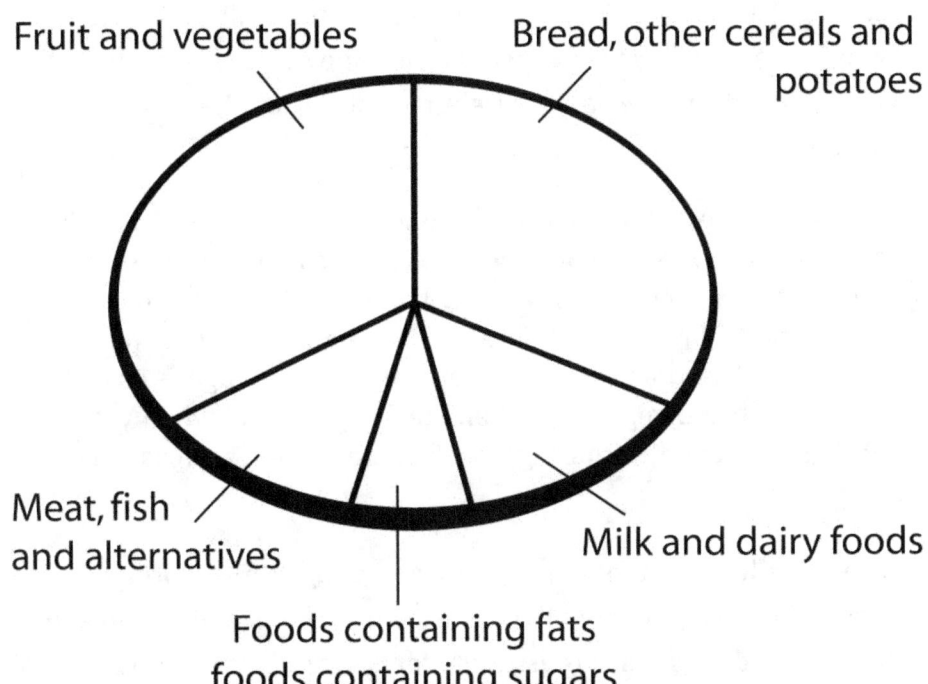

Fruit and vegetables

Bread, other cereals and potatoes

Meat, fish and alternatives

Milk and dairy foods

Foods containing fats
foods containing sugars

Diagram © food.gov.uk

This diagram represents the ideal portions of each food group we need in each meal and generally in our diets. Although it's a general guide, the principles are a good indication of what your body needs and in what quantity to function well. Weighing and portioning food isn't something I advocate – but I do meet many people who either live off fruit, or only eat carbohydrates with no protein or vegetables – who don't understand why they don't feel their best. For this reason it's important to recognise that a good balance of foods is what our bodies need. To simplify, looking at this diagram it's clear to see that you should be liberal with veg, and slightly less liberal with your protein and carbohydrate sources. It's widely accepted that supplements aren't ever a true match for getting all your nutrients from food sources – so making sure you're getting the balance right roughly is definitely important.

Most people are familiar with the concept of '5 a day' – but this appears to be ever-changing, as news articles constantly rubbish the idea then in the same breath tell us that '7 a day' is now the desired target. With vegetables again it is simple – eat as many as you want. Fruit requires more caution as it is high in sugar – so make sure you eat more vegetables than you do fruit, and when you do eat fruit, try to counter the sugar with some protein such as nuts or seeds.

Another really important part of nutrition people often forget is hydration. Drinking plenty of water each day and avoiding pop and other sugary drinks really is essential for better health – and the more vegetables you eat, the more water you'll naturally consume.

Breaking up with calories

Why counting calories is wrong

I became obsessed with counting calories when I was poorly. I'm pretty sure that many people reading this book will be obsessively counting them too, with a specific number in your mind (most probably an unreasonable one) of what constitutes your daily limit.

We are told as a guide that men should have 2,500 calories a day and women should have 2,000. This depends on activity levels, however – this is the 'base rate' needed for general bodily function and a normal level of activity. We are then told that to 'lose weight' we should consume less calories than we are expending, or in extreme circumstances less than the base rate.

The thing is, for most of us our understanding of the above is that we should be consuming as few calories as possible – regardless of what they are or where they come from. 2,000, after all, sounds like such a big number. Having this number in our heads encourages us to count. And so the obsession begins with counting, and we begin to love being in control so strongly of the little numbers in our food. A meal becomes a number of calories, fuel, not a nutritionally-balanced plate of food, as it should be.

Once you have this idea of food in your head, it's very difficult to think of it in any other way. It's hard to forget this method of thinking when at every turn you are informed of how many calories are in something or confronted with the label 'diet' or 'low calorie'. Even if you know that 'low calorie' does not in any way mean 'good for you.' I find nearly all of my friends checking the back of packets and whispering under their breath counting on their fingers when they are preparing a meal. They don't have eating disorders – they're classed as 'normal'. Sadly, this really is what is normal now.

We think of our bodies as a car, filling the car with petrol which will then be 'used up' as energy, and nothing else. However it's just not that simple – a car has lots of different elements which allow it to function properly as a whole just like the body - and therefore the fuel is then converted into different types of energy and in varying formats in order for it to work. It's not a simple 'in and out' system as we all believe.

Most types of diets 'work' (offering temporary results) because they focus on quantity and make you obsessed with calories to restrict your intake of food in general. These calorie controlled diets works for people who are morbidly obese, but most people who embark on these diets are not overweight at all – they just feel fat or are bigger than they'd like to be, unhappy with how they look.

Even though we have guidelines of calorific intake for men, women and children, everyone's 'ideal calorific intake' is different depending on age, metabolic rate, genes and activity levels, and some nutritionists even dispute whether there is an 'ideal'.

It's also worth noting that not all calories are made equal. Even though we're led to believe that we should check the number of calories in a particular item of food before we eat it, it's never explained that calories don't all behave in the same way as one another. When a calorie enters our system from one type of food, it is metabolised differently when compared with a calorie from another. This depends on a number of factors – the food the calorie is a part of, and how our bodies process it. Different people also process food differently – meaning one calorie could result in fat storage in one person but not in another. The impact is so different because the way we process food is down to our genes in part, and partly the inner health of our bodies and gut. Studies have shown that two people who exercise in the same way and eat exactly the same thing in identical amounts see different results – different levels of fat storage and different weights. This is the reason why there's really no such thing as a 'one size fits all' diet.

We're so focused on quantity - however if you get the *quality* of your food right, your body will take care of the rest.

Quality over Quantity

The more I read about nutrition and the more I looked after my body consciously as a result, the more I realised that the problems we have with food mentally (and the way to let go of those hang ups) came down to a very simple principle. I found myself quoting 'Quality over Quantity' when I spoke to people about how I ate freely and naturally and why, and how it differed from the norm. I realised that people were so concerned over the quantities of what they ate, whether that was the size of the portions themselves, the amount of meals, or the calories contained within them, that they neglected to consider the quality.

The focus for many people (and indeed of many conventional diets) is undoubtedly on quantity, when actually if the focus was on *quality,* the quantity wouldn't matter so much. I never count or weigh, I never think about my portion size, I eat when I'm hungry and I stop when I'm full. But because I concentrate on the quality of my food (plenty of vegetables, raw nuts, seeds, meat and fish) I know that my body is taking care of itself. Although I eat a lot of fat (all natural, good fats) and never count calories or worry about eating out my body hasn't changed in shape or size. I don't weigh myself, but I'm mentally and physically well enough not to care and to know that I am healthy. People are often surprised to hear that, but I know that it's because I consider Quality over Quantity.

A change in lifestyle will always feel challenging. But getting your head around Quality over Quantity is a really big first step in compounding a more balanced perspective on food.

What does 'Quality' mean? Do I have to eat organic, non GMO, gluten free, vegan or grass-fed?

I think that another confusing thing about nutrition as a concept to be followed is that the idea of what constitutes 'quality' differs between varying schools of thought. At one end of the spectrum some nutritionists and trainers would only advocate raw, unprocessed food which is free from GM and is fully organic. At the other (more realistic) end experts say that everything in moderation is fine, provided you're trying your best to source quality foods where you can. I think that in an ideal world we'd all eat organic – sourcing only natural wholefoods to eat, with grass-fed meat and dairy on the menu. But in the far from ideal world we live in most of us would never eat anything, because this type of food is hard to source expensive. It's not always feasible to eat organic or to source weird ingredients like alfalfa sprouts and spirulina powder, which is why I advocate a more balanced approach to nutrition. Where I can I eat organic food and ensure that the things I buy are responsibly sourced – but if I can't, that's okay. I wrote my recipe books to dispel the myth that eating well needs to be time-intensive and high-cost – and that proper nourishment doesn't always need to come from exclusive and expensive sources.

When I refer to 'quality' above, I mean it in a general sense. For example, a balanced, simple plate consisting of potatoes, chicken and vegetables is better quality when compared to a diet-branded ready meal. Quality doesn't need to mean expensive, organic, specialist or restrictive. It simply means that food has nutritional value and naturally associated health benefits.

Letting go of the fear of fat

I hear so many people living religiously by the phrase: 'Fat will make me 'fat'. No, it won't!

Eating fat does not make you fat – I am testament to that! Now I drink whole milk, eat butter and coconut oil and never worry about the fat content of my food. But previously I believed a 'skinny latte' made with skimmed milk was healthy, that margarine was a better alternative to butter and that I had to carefully calculate the fat contained in everything I ate because it would travel straight to my thighs as soon as it entered my mouth.

I grew up in the 90's – the decade which saw fat demonised by a relentless stream of diet 'gurus' who advised against eating any sort of fat in order to stay 'thin'. Yet fat is essential for good bodily function and is actually healthy for us in the right format and quantity. The message from diet companies is simple; as long as it is low fat, low quality and high in crap it's acceptable. But the right sort of fat is so good for you – your body needs it. Aptly-named 'good fats', such as those found in the likes of avocadoes, nuts and seeds, are not only good for your body, but also make a huge difference to your appearance. I have a diet very high in these fats and it made an indescribable difference to the health of my skin and hair. As what's on the outside is undoubtedly a reflection of what's on the inside, just think about what good fats are doing for you on the inside! Fat, in very large quantities, as with anything in excess, won't be good for you – but it is a necessary nutrient and as part of a balanced diet it is essential and beneficial for proper bodily function, providing a vital source of energy.

I remember speaking to a friend about her time at stage school in London. As a dancer, her teacher made a point of strictly controlling the students' diets in a way which would almost definitely have brought on all kinds of body-related issues. She told me that she'd only recently learned about nutrition, and that before she avoided avocado like the plague and ate chocolate instead, because this teacher had told her there was less fat in a Mars bar. I think this story really demonstrates how many people make poor choices based on a flimsy knowledge of nutrition – often passed down from others who don't understand it themselves.

Why fat is good for you

Unfortunately because the word 'fat' has negative connotations for many, actually eating it causes problems for a lot of people – especially those who have been on a variety of diets.

Despite the bad press, fat is an essential part of the human body. We need fat in our diets to aid our bodies with a number of incredibly important functions – including processes in the brain and the absorption of vitamins.

You may already have heard of Omega-3 Fatty Acids – commonly found in salmon, nuts, avocado and grass-fed meats. Because these are all foods which dieters ration due to their high fat content and high calorie count, it's likely that few of us get enough Omega-3s in our diet, which is less than good news for our bodies.

It's important to note that not all fats are good for you. Natural fats (especially those which contain Omega-3s as above) are good for you — fats which enter your mouth relatively unchanged from their raw state. However artificial fats (or trans-fats as they are also known) will never be good for you. As with all processed foods, they go through an unpalatable manufacturing process which involves chemicals and machinery before they reach your plate. Once in the body they continue to behave artificially, actively increasing bad cholesterol whilst lowering the good and causing obesity, diabetes and increased risk of heart disease. They've also been linked to some cancers. If you learn how to look after your body and follow the simple rules for health and happiness however you'll never come into contact with these fats, as they're only contained in fast foods, ready meals and processed foods.

Should I be scared of sugar?

Just as fat was demonised in the 90s, sugar has been the latest victim of panic and scrutiny along with plenty of bad press. But unlike fat, sugar has little to offer us nutritionally. Other than refined carbohydrates, there's nothing sugar can offer us or benefit us with - there are no vitamins, minerals or fibre in sugar, nor are there any anti-oxidants or helpful nutrients like fat or protein. It also disrupts the important bacteria which live in our gut and help up to absorb nutrients and digest food properly – and has even been contributed to the development of IBS and overgrowth of yeast in the intestines.

Sugar (like many things) is fine if it is consumed in moderation. However it widely recognised that most people eat too much of it - as it is now present in many of our 'staple' foods – not just in the usual suspects like cakes, sweets and biscuits. Because many people depend on processed foods they have no idea how much sugar they're consuming – especially in 'diet' foods which often replace fat with sugar. It may not always appear as 'sugar' in a list of ingredients – Fructose, Glucose and Maltose are all forms of sugar.

A lot of sugar-conscious dieters replace the sugar they can't live without with artificial sweeteners – but this isn't the answer either. Artificial, chemically-produced sweeteners like Aspartame and Sucralose (found in diet drinks, confectionery and desserts) have been found to disrupt metabolism, contribute towards cardiovascular disease and encourage weight gain in the long term. They have even been loosely linked to chronic illnesses such as cancer.

I think the bottom line with sugar (and sweeteners) is that you won't need to actively avoid it if you focus on quality foods. That's why the 'quality over quantity' mantra is a useful one – because it doesn't involve cutting out or counting – it just involves focusing on eating foods as they are supposed to be and making sure there's a benefit attached of some sort. Sugar can't be found in harmful quantities in quality foods, because they are nutritionally balanced and offer nutritional benefit.

The power of 'cheat' days

You might hear some people on diets talking about 'cheat days' – a day at the weekend where they can 'eat what they want' – usually conventionally 'unhealthy' foods in their usual form (not swaps) like pizza, crisps, chocolate and chips – without it 'wrecking their diet' or them feeling bad about it. Whilst I don't advocate this idea of a day where you can 'eat what you want' having been 'miserable' eating healthily (or worse, dieting) through the week, I do think the concept is helpful for people who are just getting used to a new way of thinking about food. Yes the name isn't particularly useful – 'cheat' implies that you are cheating on your diet and are doing something bad, but actually there's nothing wrong with eating the things which you know aren't the best for you one day a week without feeling worried about it – at least whilst you are starting to gain a more balanced view of nutrition and your body.

My justification for a cheat day here is a little unconventional – it's the concept turned on its head. So for example, you may find that whilst you get your head around the way we are supposed to eat (not worrying, weighing, controlling or limiting) you crave certain things and feel guilty and panicky about food, wanting to skip breakfast or eat a load of diet foods. Sometimes you might feel like you need relief from this new way of thinking. That's where cheat days come in – let your insecurities back in and give them space for just a day or half a day until you don't feel as though you need a 'cheat' day anymore.

This is a day where anything goes. When I was first getting my head around nutrition I started with cheat days every Saturday – days when I might not eat properly, stuffed my face with the sugary things I'd lived off before or skipped breakfast just because I needed a release, even though I knew that it was wrong. I'd reserve this day for meals out too. Eventually, I stopped wanting or needing cheat days and now I just eat the in the same way every single day without thinking about it, never feeling bad about food or worrying about my weight, eating out whenever I want to. Nobody makes a significant change in belief and behaviour overnight, which is why I believe 'cheat' days can be helpful at first, even though they should not become a habit or a sustained way of living.

80/20

A good way to help yourself to adopt a balanced view when it comes to nutrition is to remember the 80/20 concept – another thing I find myself saying a lot when I speak to people about how they eat. You might be familiar with the idea that good health and a healthy body is achieved 80% through nutrition, 20% exercise (this has certainly been my experience, although it is often debated), but I also want to introduce another side of 80/20.

Numbers and food together for me are usually a no-no, but for those just starting out on their nutrition journey there are a couple of reasons why 80/20 is a useful principle to keep in mind where nutrition is concerned. Along with Quality over Quantity this can help you to develop and maintain a healthier attitude towards food without feeling worried or deprived.

The idea with this is that most of the time (roughly 80%) you eat as you know you should (not thinking about what you eat, choosing wholesome food, not giving in to a 'diet' mentality), then 20% of the time you have that cake if you don't want to swap it, have a few drinks and a fast food burger a load of sweets, skip breakfast etc. Eventually 80% will become 100%, as it is for me now.

The 'all or nothing' mentality 'cutting out' and 'counting' diets promote causes us to crave control and dismiss responsible advice, not feeling comfortable with the concept of balance and sensible eating – which is why it's so hard to shake off that feeling that you will suddenly become 'fat', feel incredibly anxious when you don't monitor, weigh or count – or panic when you introduce a food group you'd been avoiding for so long. Once you feel you don't need 'cheat days' or that '20%', you know you are well on your way to maintaining a healthy relationship with food.

6. Mythbusters

It's great to see that increasingly nutritionists, trainers and dieticians are 'de-bunking' common food myths to help us all to live more healthily. However these less sensationalistic pieces of information are often not publicised quite as much as the 'FAST FOR A DAY A WEEK AND LOSE A STONE' or 'RED MEAT IS ACTUALLY GOOD FOR YOU' headlines. Often carefully-conducted, official (scientifically and medically correct) research is manipulated by the press, which is what leads to confusing and often directly contradictory articles we find in newspapers and magazines (sometimes both in one edition!)

It's worrying and frustrating that so many vulnerable people believe these articles - and compromise their health unknowingly as a result. It's absolutely a prominent driver behind so many people's distorted view of food and the consequential health crises we're experiencing in the Western world.

Although it's not possible for me to cover absolutely every piece of irresponsible nonsense in the book, I've included a few common ones below with reasons why they are far from the truth. Some of the information might seem repetitive given previous chapters, but this should hopefully serve as a quick guide to flick through if you ever feel as though you're doubting yourself of feel fearful over food again.

Remember that whatever you may have heard or believed before, in this book you'll only find a factual, balanced view.

MYTH: Carbs will make me 'fat'

Low-carb diets have always been popular, mostly because they do very quickly result in weight loss (remember that weight is just a number, and that 'weight loss' alone isn't necessarily a good thing). But carbohydrate alone will not make you fat, contrary to what certain diet companies, celebrities and magazines will have you believe. These diets work because carbohydrates (being a good source of energy) tend to have lots of calories in them gram for gram, so limiting these (and therefore limiting calories) results in weight loss. Eating carbohydrates as part of a balanced diet will not make you 'fat' or cause you to put on weight.

MYTH: I can 'exercise off' food or 'burn off' calories

When I'm at the gym I often hear people saying *'I'm working off last night's curry'* or *'I'm working off that biscuit'.* Indeed this is the principle I lived by when I was poorly and for some time after; I'd calculate how many calories I'd consumed and then try to work them all off that same evening by calculating how many calories the exercise would 'use up'. I was then 'neutral'; in my head I'd consumed nothing, it had been a good day. As I got older I lived by the same principle – even though I technically was free of an eating disorder, my habits still revolved around calories, and limiting or 'burning' them off.

Evidently this was harmful and wrong in so many ways. But even in a less extreme example than with Anorexia or very disordered eating, like those people at the gym, it's a wholly inaccurate representation of the way our bodies work. Looking at calories as fuel is helpful, but not a description that should be taken in completely the same way as how a car or an aeroplane might use fuel. Your body is working constantly. Have you ever heard that our bodies repair themselves when we are asleep? That we consume a fair amount of energy even though we are lying down?

The idea that you have a number going in and therefore have to have a number going out is completely irrational. It's not just about the number, it is about what you eat, the nutrients contained within that food, how easily, quickly, slowly it is digested, what it is used for once it is in your body.

It comes back down to the simplification of nutrition - the idea that it's just about the numbers of what goes in (and what goes out) and not about the content or the *quality* of what you eat. Your body uses food in lots of different ways, at varying times and in different amounts. It uses food as fuel, for lots of different functions, not just 'burning it' through sheer activity.

MYTH: If I eat like a certain person and exercise like a certain person, I will look like that person

That there are so many articles out there documenting what a particular celebrities eats and how they work out, encouraging people to emulate that so they can 'look like them'. The harmful (and frankly irresponsible) message this gives to women and especially to younger people is 'if you do this...you'll look like that'.

From person to person, metabolism, shape, size and weight are all different. There are so many variables that make you who you are. No diet will change that. Nobody ever told me this – I took what magazines told me as gospel. I followed diet plans endorsed by celebrities who were nearly 6ft tall with naturally long, slim legs. Even though I followed the diet religiously, my legs didn't look like theirs - because I am 5'4" and my thighs and bum are the biggest parts of me! I didn't know that at the time though, of course. I couldn't understand why, in my opinion, I was still 'fat' and 'dumpy' and disliked. Even if you were to select a celebrity who is the same body type and height as you, you are still two different people. Once I learned about metabolism I longed for a fast one because I was told that that's what slim people had. But once again that's not necessarily true. It's not always possible (or a good thing) to 'speed up' your metabolism – and schemes like this almost certainly come under the 'diet' umbrella, which (as mentioned previously) are harmful for all sorts of reasons and actually wreck your natural metabolism in the long run.

MYTH: I have to count calories and fat and sugar religiously otherwise I will be fat

This is the biggest myth of all. There are SO many people who lay a lot of store by counting calories. Checking packets, asking friends if they know, worrying if it's over a certain number. Perhaps you're one of them. But as I say throughout this book, as long as you're eating the right food, in reasonable quantities, your body will sort itself out and so will your weight, whether you're going up or down the scale. Counting calories and fat religiously causes us to become abnormally concerned (obsessed even) with controlling what we eat – and in many cases that can cause people to continue in a vicious cycle of eating too much, because they are always so focused on food. At the other end of the spectrum it can lead to an eating disorder, or at best a miserable life spent adding and subtracting.

MYTH: There is a perfect way to eat

Even some of the most prestigious dieticians can advocate a 'perfect' way of eating, but many will tell you that there simply isn't one 'perfect' way to eat. Not only is everybody different, but even looking at it from an individual perspective, there isn't a particular amount, or variation, or even time to eat which should be followed scrupulously, with 'catastrophic' results if not. It's about balance, and unfortunately for the diet-induced control freak in you, it's pretty vague in principle. You are healthy as long as you eat a good balanced natural diet. It's that simple.

MYTH: Fat is bad for you

This is something I've already covered in detail – but it's one of the most widely-believed nutrition myths. Fat is essential and should be included in your diet – especially if you want to keep your body fit and healthy. You can find sources of 'good fat' in dairy products, certain vegetables, meats, fish, nuts and seeds. Just remember to steer clear of processed trans-fats which are present in junk foods, ready meals and snacks.

MYTH: There are 'Good' and 'Bad' foods

I always understood that some foods were okay to eat all the time, and some weren't so good. For instance, I understood quite early on that I could have as many vegetables as I wanted, but we only ever had McDonald's occasionally. I knew there was a reason behind that - the food I could have more of was better for me. It wasn't until later that I believed that foods were grouped into two categories – 'good' and 'bad'. Which category a particular item fell into depended largely on the school of thought or particular diet advice I'd been given, but generally it followed the rules we all live by – chips are 'bad', spinach is 'good'. Water is 'good', fizzy drinks are 'bad'. It's ironic to think that as children we probably have a more rounded view of food and we care much less – but that in lots of ways our opinions are formed then and as we enter our teens, when we become more aware of how we look and have more control over what we eat.

As adults we're often encouraged to make 'all or nothing' style dietary sacrifices - to avoid a certain thing completely, or cut out certain food groups. It's this sort of mentality which causes people to have an unhealthy relationship with food – one where we are obsessed with 'good' and 'bad' and counting calories and cutting things out. Why do foods have to be grouped into 'bad' and 'good'? This categorisation of food only serves to further alienate us from it and allows us too much choice and control over what we eat. It demonises certain foods and therefore makes it easier to limit and control, actively encouraging us to eliminate food groups and foods because we think that they are 'bad'. Diet companies persuade you to do this because it looks like an easy 'quick fix' to weight loss – because of course you are cutting out a whole food group or portion of your diet. It's no different from slimming pills which make you go to the toilet – it's phantom weight loss and it's the worst thing you can do to your body.

MYTH: 'Diet', 'natural' and 'low fat' is good for you

For me, a container with 'diet' or 'low-fat' on it is a good reason to avoid whatever's inside it. That's because these foods have been modified and messed with to appear healthier. This might be fine if they actually offered tangible benefits either for sensible weight loss or sustained health – but in actual fact they do the opposite.

Yoghurts are one of the best examples of this. Diet yoghurts claim to be a healthy alternative to 'real' (full-fat) yoghurt – yet manufacturers have tampered with the raw dairy product to remove fat, then replace the fat with sugar, sweeteners, preservatives and colourings. Even those which claim to be 'natural' or 'organic' will have some form of added sugar in them.

What this means is that you replace a wholesome, all-natural yoghurt filled with good bacteria, healthy fat and nutrients (not to mention low in sugar) with an artificial product which has been made in a factory and contains more sugar than chocolate (some 'light' or 'diet' branded yoghurts contain 16-18g of sugar – more than a Cadbury's Dairy Milk bar).

Cereals are also good example of this – and healthy 'protein' bars. A leading diet cereal brand has more sugar in it than some of its chocolatey counterparts aimed at children.

Whether it's a ready meal or a cereal bar, remember that what you are eating has been processed. It might be 'low-fat', but it can simultaneously be high in sugar and salt which are equally (if not more) bad for you. This is the only 'label checking' I'd condone – because really, the best foods come without labels and long lists of ingredients.

MYTH: Quick fixes work

We've all heard the phrase 'too good to be true'. It's a good motto to keep in mind when considering diets, because our bodies are not designed to accommodate quick fixes. They expect us to look after them consistently with a constant stream of quality nutrients and sufficient nourishment so that they can function properly. Messing up that finely-balanced equilibrium can have many negative consequences which you may never even see – but you might feel the subtle difference – a lack of energy, lethargy, irritability, dry skin, hair loss, stomach issues.

The only way to be healthy and to lose weight (if you need to) is to do so safely and slowly. If you really do need to lose weight, then investing the money you'd have spent on a diet in the advice of a qualified nutritionist or dietician is the best thing you can do. Exercise is also important. If you hate the thought of the gym or running, how about starting off walking, cycling, swimming or attending a dance class?

I know that for many people a 'quick fix' is too attractive to resist – it's human nature to be impatient and it's especially important to feel as though the things which make you feel bad about yourself and any perceived imperfections can be rapidly fixed or eradicated. But doing things the right way is beneficial for you in so many ways. Self-esteem is also important – so if you are stuck in a damaging cycle of serial dieting and don't feel able to see your way out, it's worth addressing your self-esteem first (there's more about this in Tough Love).

MYTH: Diet pills are a good idea

Please, please, please never take diet pills. I can't stress this enough.

Diet pills are never a good idea. If they worked, or if they were a healthy long-term alternative to eating responsibly and exercising, GPs would prescribe them. Doctors and consultants would advise obese people to take them if they were a viable and safe method of sustained weight loss. But they're not.

Most 'over the counter' diet pills or 'detox powders' are a form of laxative. Whether you're 12 stone or 20, if you have diarrhoea for a few days on the run, you're bound to see the number on the scales go down. That's because your stomach and bowels are consistently empty.

Diet pills deprive you of nutrients, dehydrate you and confuse your gut. They're bad news all round – but especially if you find them on the internet. So many needless deaths have been caused by people taking pills they've sourced from the internet with questionable origins – it's simply not worth it, however 'fat' you feel and however unhappy you are with your body. There is an alternative – and you can find more details about this at the back of the book.

Myth: Unconventional diets are better for me

Whilst many of the principles of 'paleo', 'caveman' and 'raw' diets mirror the advice I offer here in this book, they are *still diets*. This means that you're still cutting out, rationing or limiting some type of food. Often they can lead to an obsession with food quality (sometimes known as Orthorexia) – meaning you become 'afraid' of anything which is not raw, organic, 'gluten free' or 'vegan'. Whilst these diets may be slightly better than the conventional regimes, they are still trends which can be harmful and aren't necessarily good for you if they're in place for any sustained length of time.

7. My perspective – how I eat and why I eat this way

This is not a book about me telling you how you should eat and what you should do – but I thought it would be helpful to share my perspective now and the types of food I make sure I include in my diet to be as healthy as possible.

Before

I talk in previous chapters a little bit about the way I was before, because I want you to know that I was just like you. Maybe I was better, maybe I was worse – but the one thing we have in common is the warped, false idea of food and the role it plays in our lives.

Everyone knows that eating disorders are bad news. I was lucky enough to 'recover' from mine to a point where I did have a healthier relationship with food – at least for a few years. But I never developed a healthier relationship with myself – or my body. I still didn't feel good enough, slim enough, pretty enough. I suffered with body dysmorphia and as a result my obsession with food started to creep back in. So although I never relapsed and developed Anorexia again, I picked up some bad habits and started to revolve my life around the way I looked, which I see now was a recipe for unhappiness.

At the time, it seemed like the only way to be happy – to have everything I wanted. I still equated looking good in the eyes of others to being liked, so this was important to me, even though I was aware of how superficial it was. From the age of 16 to the age of 22, I spent a lot of time considering how I could change myself aesthetically. I was turned down for cosmetic surgery. I spent all my money on make-up, hair extensions and beauty products, and spent all my time worrying about being 'good enough'. Part of this of course involved my body – and that involved food.

I spent a lot of my earlier years after college working in various retail jobs. The long, sometimes anti-social hours and a lengthy commute left me with little choice but to eat on the go (usually one apple here and there) – but that suited me. It meant I had little time to think about food or eat it.

Working 12 hour days standing in heels I'd have an apple or a cereal bar for breakfast and a cup soup for lunch. I'd go home and have a meal, but none of it was enough to sustain me – and the calorie and fat content had all been carefully counted. I ate pretty much the same thing every single day – fearful of deviating in case I piled on the pounds. I weighed myself once a week every Friday, feeling sick with dread in case I'd gained a pound. I loved being thin and conveniently dismissed the low energy levels, brittle nails, irritability and poor skin condition. After all, these symptoms were nothing compared to what I'd been through with Anorexia.

Following my time in retail I eventually got a desk job. This involved little activity – cue the anxiety in my head over where I would 'burn off' my calories. It was harder too to limit food, as I was sat all day long thinking about it with little to distract me or stop me from grabbing my lunch from the fridge. I became obsessed with finding a new way to eat to suit my new lifestyle, but just as I did, I found I struggled to eat certain things and ended up only eating sweets and sugary things. I was diagnosed with IBS – and I felt miserable about being unable to eat so many things. I wondered whether there was a cure or treatment - then started to research online. Then I ended up at the gym and realised I needed to eat more. Because I wasn't able to, I relied on branded diet marshmallow wafers to get me through the day, eating two packets just to have the energy to meet clients and do my job properly. Although this all seems to be about food, the root of my behaviour was my low self-esteem. Everything I ate was carefully calculated to ensure I didn't get 'fat' – a fear I'd held for a very long time.

Self-esteem is something which can be improved with time and the right tools and guidance. I wrote Tough Love to support people going through the same thing I did just a couple of years ago – and I go into a lot more detail about body image and improving that there. The focus of this book though is food – and just from the small excerpt of my story above you've probably got the idea that me and food weren't friends. In fact the less I ate the better. So how did I change that around, why did I change, and how has it benefitted me?

What about now?

I try as closely as possible to eat the way I feel I was 'supposed to eat'. That's whole, natural, unprocessed foods. My recipe books are all about simple, wholesome recipes which are inexpensive to make and most importantly of all which taste amazing. I'm not about spending hours in the kitchen or sprouting beans for days – I'm **real**. I'm a real person with a very busy lifestyle – plus I don't have hundreds of pounds to spend every month on food. Instead I devised my own easy, simplistic and tasty recipes and tried to include as many nutritious ingredients in each as I could.

Although I've been told that the way I eat is similar to 'raw' 'paleo' and 'clean-eating' diets, I don't recommend or endorse any particular sort of 'diet' – because that's not what I believe in. What I do believe in is that healthy eating shouldn't be temporary, it should be for life. All you have to do is be honest and eat healthy, wholesome food, drink plenty of water – and your body will take care of itself. What I wanted to do was to find a way to eat that was better for my body and didn't harm my health, without depriving myself, starving myself or feeling miserable.

After years of abuse (though I wasn't aware of the harmful effects I would suffer at the time) I'm eating much better and I do see the physical benefits of that – some of which counteract the after-effects I still struggle with now following Anorexia and years of poor nutrition.

When I've introduced other people to my way of eating, they have seen a dramatic improvement in their health. Some have even lost weight – just by eating naturally the way they always should have done. Often they tell me they can't believe that eating without thinking and having full-fat everything could achieve results like this, but I always say 'it's just the way we were meant to be.' One thing's for sure – they also tell me how miserable they were throughout their years of dieting, and how much happier they are now being able to live their lives free from the shackles of counting, agonising and panicking over how they eat.

My Superfoods

These aren't all 'superfoods' in the conventional sense – some of them are actually very ordinary. But they're my superfoods because I feel they have made a significant difference since I've included them in my diet and they're things that everyone can easily incorporate and enjoy.

Something which annoys me (and is often brought to my attention) is the high cost of eating healthily. Often we pay a premium for food in its raw state – for example, salted nuts are cheaper than raw nuts. How does that make sense? Although the supermarkets have got things the wrong way round, it *is* possible to eat well on a budget. Vegetables, nuts and quality dairy products can be found relatively cheaply at budget supermarkets and world food stores – and butchers and fishmongers aren't always as expensive as you might think.

There are so many foods I eat on a daily and weekly basis – I just couldn't include them all here. But I've tried to cut it down to the real superstars and things which I eat often – with added information and vital statistics on why they are so beneficial. If you're reading this book with a 'diet company' mentality, some of these may surprise you! They're *real* foods. If you fancy trying some of these and are struggling for inspiration, take a look at my recipe books *(there's more information on these in Chapter 10 of this book).*

Coconut – Everyone who knows me knows I love all things coconut. Happily for me and any other coconut lovers out there, coconut is actually very good for us and its various products each have wonderful health benefits attached to them. Originally I started using desiccated coconut in my food and then began to use coconut oil and coconut flour in my baking.

Fast forward a couple of years, and coconut has recently been hailed a superfood. With that, many products have seen increased popularity. Coconut oil and coconut flour are now widely used and are much more readily available.

Coconut has such a wide range of benefits for the body in all its forms. Coconut oil in particular is a good all-rounder for the body because it is rich in fatty acids and is a good source of energy as well as containing Lauric Acid, which has lots of different uses in the body but notably helps maintain healthy skin and hair. It also helps to look after your digestive tract as it has anti-microbial pro-biotic properties which keep stomach nasties and yeast at bay.

Coconut is really versatile – meaning there's lots of different by-products. Here are a few I use below, what they are and how you can use them.

Coconut Water

Coconut water is what you can hear sloshing around inside a coconut – but the type you drink comes from a young coconut which is softer and green – not the matured brown hairy variety. It's rich in electrolytes (which aid hydration) and naturally sweet, yet fairly low in sugar. The best way to enjoy coconut water is straight out of a fresh young green coconut – but unfortunately we don't have that luxury in the UK – so you're more likely to find it in your local supermarket. There are lots of different varieties of coconut water now, some with added fruit pulps which are very nice. I like Unoco as it tastes fresh, delicious and is completely raw – plus you can mix it into 'cocktails' as I do in the book for a healthy refreshing treat.

Coconut Oil

I use coconut oil a lot for baking and also have a spoonful every morning with my breakfast. It has a distinctive sweet coconut flavour – some people use it in savoury dishes but I only like it for sweet recipes. Along with coconut water, coconut oil was arguably the first coconut product to receive renowned nutritional status. Most large supermarkets now sell cold-pressed, organic coconut oil fairly cheaply but Coconoil, Lucy Bee, Biona and Tiana are all good quality brands which can be found online.

Coconut Butter

Coconut butter is similar to coconut oil but is less greasy and has the same relationship to coconut oil as olive oil spread might have to olive oil. I use coconut butter in baking and for making raw chocolate – it has a less strong coconut flavour than the oil but is rich and creamy. I like Biona Coconut Bliss – but Tiana also do lots of different types of oils and butters some with added Omega 3.

Coconut Flour

Coconut flour is essentially dried milled coconut meat which takes a powdery flour-like form. It's higher in protein than its counterparts and is also rich in fibre as well as having some of the other antioxidant and nutritional benefits of coconut. It's really versatile and great for baking; it has a sweet slightly coconutty taste so if I don't want to make a coconut-flavoured dish I usually mix it with almond or rice flour.

Coconut Palm Sugar

Coconut palm sugar or 'palm sugar' comes from the sap of flowers from the coconut palm tree. It looks like brown sugar and similarly has a rich caramel flavour which makes it perfect for toffee and caramel dishes – but for that reason it's not always suitable for lighter desserts. I use organic coconut sugar.

Flaked or Desiccated Coconut

The most familiar form of coconut in western diets until its emergence as a popular health food, the older generations will be familiar with desiccated coconut from ice buns and coconut ice sweets. It is made from dried coconut meat which is then flaked either into tiny pieces or larger shavings.

As well as using coconut extensively in my cooking, I also use coconut oil to moisturise my hair and skin – plus it's great as a lip balm.

Avocado – It's not everyone's thing - but if you love avocado that's good news, because your body loves it too. Unfortunately avocado got side-lined recently because of its high fat content – but the fats that avocadoes contain are actually *good* for you. I often have avocado with smoked salmon or in salads – it's really versatile and some people even make desserts with it. The best bit nutritionally is the darker green flesh right under the skin – so make sure you peel instead of chopping so you don't miss out on it.

Avocado is a superfood for me because it's really nutrient dense, full of good things for the body. Even a small serving provides good amounts of vitamins K, C, B5, B6 and E – plus Magnesium, Iron, Potassium Zinc, Thiamin, Riboflavin and Niacin. That's without mentioning that avocadoes are full of healthy mono- and poly-unsaturated fats and Omega-3s, which are good for the body as a whole but especially the heart, in addition to high amounts of fibre which make them easily digestible.

Nuts – Nuts are incredible. Each type is different in texture, flavour and size – yet all are packed full of healthy nutrients and vitamins. Remember to always try to have nuts raw where you can – as they're not so good for you after they've been coated with salt, monosodium glutamate and other nasties.

Almonds, cashews and pistachios contain Omega 3 Fatty Acids (great for healthy hair, nails, skin), protein and fibre (which helps keep you full). Peanuts are full of Vitamin E and folate which is vital for brain development and foetal development in pregnant women. Brazil nuts – one of my personal favourites – are packed with selenium and good fats.

My main reason for eating nuts is their nutritious qualities for skin and hair. I notice a big difference if I go without them or don't substitute them in my diet. They're also really tasty and full of energy so I always have them handy as a snack when I'm on the go.

Nuts are also versatile. As I am gluten intolerant I often use almond flour in baking – and nut butters for chocolate-like sweet snacks.

There really is no need to be confused about nuts. Some people avoid them as they are high in calories and fat, yet just like avocadoes, the type of fat they contain is *good* for us. They are also similar to any other food in that in moderation, they are fine to eat and considering they're filled with added nutrients, why wouldn't you include them in your diet?

Eggs - Often overlooked as a 'staple' grocery – we consume 11.7 billion each year in the UK – that's 32 million per day. Eggs are incredibly versatile – plus they are light and suitable for people who are poorly or have digestive issues. Packed with protein in addition to Selenium, Iron, Vitamin D and a host of B-Vitamins, they really are a fantastic addition to any diet.

I have eggs at least once a week – I either bake them into a soufflé or quiche and I'll often have them poached with salmon in a salad, or scrambled or devilled as a snack.

Cocoa – We constantly see headlines telling us that chocolate is 'good for us' – but many think 'how could that possibly be?' That's because the *cocoa* in chocolate is filled with antioxidant properties and unique nutrients. Chocolate is something many of us love – but know to be 'bad' for us. The reason for this is that chocolate in its usual form has been processed and has had extra fat added, as well as lots of sugar. It's these added things which make conventional chocolate products something to eat in moderation – however the good news is that you can make your own chocolatey treats which don't feature added sugars, meaning you can enjoy them whenever you like.

Cocoa, the main ingredient in chocolate, is actually incredibly good for us. Cacao (the proper name for it in its raw state) contains Polyphenols, which have been shown to protect the heart and maintain healthy blood flow. Cacao also has a positive effect on mood – as it boosts two 'feel good' chemicals in the brain – serotonin and dopamine. You may have heard of serotonin, as some anti-depressants are known as SSRIs or 'Selective Seratonin Re-uptake Inhibitors'. Cocoa has also been said to help with digestive complaints as it encourages the growth of good bacteria in the gut – another welcome benefit.

Outside of the kitchen cocoa powder can be used in a hair mask to help hair loss – and you'll probably already know that raw cocoa butter is great for moisturising skin and hair. Raw, organic Cacao is the best form of cocoa to use as it is not roasted, therefore retaining the antioxidant qualities better – however I do sometimes use Bourneville or Green and Black's. To experience the full benefit of Cacao you can try the chocolate recipes in my recipe books.

Fish – We all know that fish is good for us. Salmon, tuna, sardines, cod, prawns – whichever type of seafood takes your fancy, it's bound to have some fabulous benefits for your body. Salmon especially is a nutritionist's favourite because of its rich combination of healthy attributes. Aside from being dense in Omega-3 and unique amino acids, they are high in protein and contain vitamins such as Selenium, Biotin and Vitamins B-12 and D, which all play vital roles in many of our bodily functions. Where possible, try to eat as many different parts of the fish as you can. I even love to eat salmon skin if it's crispy. Sardines and anchovies are great for this reason because you eat the whole fish, obtaining all the benefits of the little bones and connective tissue which you would normally miss out on when eating larger fish fillets.

Greens – Whilst it's important to include a range of different coloured veg in your diet, green vegetables are fantastic for overall health which is why they get a special mention here. Dark, leafy green veg (such as spinach, kale and certain types of lettuce), are packed with vitamins and minerals. They also contain a high amount of Phytochemicals (or anti-oxidants) and fibre which gives your digestive system a helping hand.

Dairy – I believe that unless you are lactose intolerant, there is no reason not to eat dairy products or exclude them from your diet. Whole milk, like butter, has been tossed out in favour of skimmed milk, which is actually a lot less healthy. Whole milk isn't high fat at all nutritionally-speaking – plus its added vitamins A, D, E and K can't be found in the same quantities in skimmed varieties. Greek yoghurt is another star of the dairy category. Filled with important gut-loving probiotics and rich in protein, it's the perfect accompaniment at breakfast, lunch and dinner given its versatile taste and texture. Unprocessed cheeses are also good for us – contributing to healthy gut flora and even aiding weight maintenance.

I could go on forever about dairy - cream, crème fraiche, fromage frais, sour cream and cheese – they're all incredibly good for you and as with anything, are great consumed as part of a balanced diet.

Butter – I know that butter is technically dairy, but really it does deserve a little piece all of its own. Back in the 80s and 90s (and ever since, actually) butter has been portrayed as the devil's food by many a diet company, especially following the 'low fat' revolution. They'll tell you that processed margarines made from congealed oils (AKA trans fats) are the way forward - however pure, unsalted butter is not at all a sadistic fat-monster as diet companies will have you believe. It's been a staple part of our diets for many years and in some recipes, such as my sticky toffee pudding, butter adds unrivalled richness and flavour. Grass-fed butter and ghee in particular contain a potent mix of omega-3s and -6s, in addition to vitamins and EFAs (Essential Fatty Acids).

Spices and Herbs – Often the bits and bobs we add to our food can be overlooked – but in actual fact these powerful flavoursome additions can have an extra positive effect on our health by their inclusion in our diets. Herbs have been used to create medicines for thousands of years – so it's no surprise that sage has been shown to boost memory and reduce inflammation, rosemary has been found to ease stress and soothe indigestion, and thyme has proven anti-bacterial properties. For savoury dishes, I love cayenne pepper (for digestion and circulation), cumin (high in iron and helps liver to detox) and turmeric (powerful anti-inflammatory and antioxidant qualities as well as benefits for the brain and mental health, including depression). On the sweet side, I love to add cinnamon and ginger to my food – not only are they warm, spicy flavours, but cinnamon aids digestion and aids circulation, ginger also helps with digestion and reduces inflammation, and both boast antioxidant properties.

Collagen and Gelatine – I always used to think gelatine was a bit disgusting, and not without reason – for those who don't know, it's a by-product of meat made from the bones and less desirable bits of animals. However now I know how good it can be for you, I make it an important part of my diet.

I have collagen (made by Great Lakes) every day in powder form (collagen hydrolysate) mixed into my breakfast, and if I can I also mix it into other meals, too. It's tasteless and dissolves completely in food and liquid unlike gelatine, which sets and jellifies your food. Collagen helps to repair and restore many different parts of our bodies – such as bones, cartilage, skin, hair and tendons. You might have heard of collagen before in an advert for an expensive face cream, and their claims of a 'youthful glow' attributed to collagen are half-right. As it is only absorbed when consumed through eating the bone marrow, cartilage and skin of animals, we're unfortunately missing out on a lot of the collagen we could and should have because we just don't eat those things anymore.

Including additional collagen in your diet provides your body with additional amino acids which build connective tissue and regulate and maintain vital cell functions. This is so important for anybody really, given the lack of collagen in modern diets – but especially anyone recovering from Anorexia or any chronic illness. Not only will your skin, hair and nails thank you, the rest of your body will too.

Sweet Freedom – I never feel it's reasonable to expect anyone (especially sugar fiends) to go 'cold turkey' – and this is my secret weapon both in baking and for those who drink tea and coffee. Sweet Freedom is made from a blend of carob and fruit sugars, so it is low GI and low in glucose. It tastes great in cakes, biscuits and sauces and is my alternative to coconut palm sugar in recipes which demand a lighter sugar.

Oats - A pretty unremarkable, boring-looking superfood. Without the snazzy bright colours which blueberries and beetroots boast, they are admittedly a little bit beige - not the most exciting colour. But there's nothing boring about the benefits that oats boast for your body.

I love oats – they're the main component in porridge and flapjacks which I have often, and I sometimes use oats in my cakes and cookies. They're really versatile as a food and because they aren't overpoweringly flavoured, they're a great base to add whatever toppings you fancy to.

Porridge, home-made granola and flapjacks are great breakfast choices - I love plain oats or chocolate oats made with whole milk to make them creamy.

Oats are high in fibre and protein, so they're good for energy and digestion. They also contain good amounts of Manganese, a mineral which supports skin, hair and bone health – as well as iron and a host of other vitamins, minerals and antioxidants. Because you're unlikely to consume oats dry, you're also getting the added benefit of yoghurt or milk and the toppings you choose – like berries and nuts. If you buy them in their raw state they're also 100% natural – so what's not to like?

Seeds – Like nuts, seeds may be little but they pack a powerful punch nutritionally-speaking. There are so many different types of seeds – so you're bound to find one that you like. They don't all behave in the same way, either - you may have heard recently about in-vogue superfood chia seeds, which 'puff up' to make pudding-style desserts and healthy porridge-style breakfasts. All seeds have health benefits – but there are a few which are especially notable, like pumpkin seeds and flaxseed. The flaxseed (or linseed) you'll find in shops is the golden milled powder created when the indigestible husks of the seeds are removed. Flaxseed is high in fibre and omega-3 essential fatty acids making it the perfect addition to any meal – I sprinkle it over salads, bake it into cakes and cookies and mix it in with Greek yoghurt in the morning. Like nut oils, seed oils are also really popular additions to diets and contain similar health benefits to the seeds themselves.

Rapeseed Oil – I use cold-pressed Rapeseed Oil in my savoury cooking for frying, coating and also in baking for certain cakes and cookies. It has a really light flavour and is golden yellow in colour. Rapeseed Oil is rich in Vitamin E and healthy mono-unsaturated fats and has a high smoke point (meaning it retains its nutrients at very high temperatures) which makes it a more nutritious alternative for cooking with when compared to Olive Oil.

Pulses – Pulses include beans, lentils and peas. They are high in fibre and protein and some contain vital nutrients, vitamins and minerals including iron, magnesium and B vitamins. I often use gram flour (made from chickpeas) as it's gluten-free and high in protein and fibre – plus it's incredibly tasty and versatile enough to use in a range of dishes to make breads, batters and patties. Make sure you find pulses dried or if you use tinned pulses ensure they have nothing added to them such as salt, sugar or preservatives.

If you need inspiration and tips on incorporating these superfoods into your diet, you can find my downloadable recipe books at **www.toughcookieblog.co.uk.**

8. Taking the first steps to better nutrition

In lots of ways you have already taken the first step to better nutrition – by reading this book! Hopefully now you will have a clearer understanding of how food can help you and should be enjoyed rather than demonised. However just reading one book doesn't change the habits of a lifetime – and it's likely you'll find yourself continuing to avoid fat, checking packets and counting calories sometimes. That's okay – because nobody stops doing something they've done for a long time just like that.

The key now is to recognise when you are doing that, put the packet down and walk away. Eventually, you won't even bother to pick it up anymore. In fact, it's best to eat foods which don't come in packets with ingredients lists and nutritional information at all – so when you go shopping, try to have as many things in your trolley in their recognisable state as possible – fruit and vegetables, meats, fish, nuts, eggs and cheeses. Stay away from diet food completely and make everything from scratch as opposed to buying processed foods – even if they say 'natural' on them.

I know that lots of people are way too busy to 'make everything from scratch'. I'm busy too! I *have* to make sure my food is prepared in advance due to my Irritable Bowel Syndrome – because there's simply nothing I can eat otherwise. That's why I make a lot in bulk, and store chillis, curries and stews in my freezer ready for when I simply don't have time or can't be bothered. It *can* be done – especially if you develop a few key favourite recipes which are quick and easy to make – like cheese grilled over beef tomatoes or omelette or chicken kebabs.

It's important whilst you're making changes not to be hard on yourself – just do the best you can. I hope this book has shown you that nutrition is not about 'don't do this, don't eat that' – it's about being as healthy as you possibly can be with the right motives behind you – enjoying food without worrying about it or overthinking it. Take one step at a time – this doesn't have to be a dramatic overnight change. The fact that you are making a conscious effort to change is all that matters. Lots of people underestimate the positive impact small lifestyle changes can have – just walking instead of getting in the car, taking the stairs instead of the lift and swapping your usual mid-morning cereal bar for a healthier alternative. Slowly but surely implementing these small changes to habit can help you to live more healthily.

Lastly, once you've read this book and implemented some of the new information you've discovered, keep learning. I wrote this book in a simple, easy to understand way – so there's a lot more you could get to know about food and nutrition. If you're curious like I was, you'll be able to find lots of studies, papers and blogs online which discuss nutrition in a scientific and factual way. It's an interesting and extensive subject and as with everything, knowledge is power – the more you know and understand about your body and the way it works, the less likely you'll be to get drawn in again by a fad diet or tempted to question your new approach in favour of a 'quick fix'.

If you're struggling for inspiration and haven't already purchased my recipe books, you can see details of these at the back of this book – and if you need further support with self-esteem or body image you can read more about Tough Love in the *'Further Reading'* chapter.

9. The last word

I always try to include three, easy to remember take away messages in each of my books. That way if you ever feel as though you need a boost or a reminder, you can flick to the back and take a look through these for inspiration.

1/ *Your body is **amazing***

Your body is an incredible thing. You use it all day, every day – it never stops working, but you probably take it for granted. Take time to consider that when you skip a meal, eat rubbish food or starve yourself, you are hurting your body. You might not think that it has any significant effect, but I can tell you first hand that in the long term it will. There is nothing more important than your health – without that, you can't live your life the way you want to, do the things you want to do. Always remember (especially when tempted to take diet pills or sign up to a new regime) that your body and your health should always come first.

2/ ***Diets are bad for you*** *– full stop*

Often people come to me and say *'You know, the one I'm on isn't that bad – you can eat what you want'* or *'it's changed now – you can eat a lot more.'* My answer is still the same though – it's a diet, it's temporary, it's irresponsible and it won't work in the long-term. It involves tracking your weight, thinking about food more than you would normally, and they take your money for the privilege.

They'll always be the same – and they'll ever be good for you. Don't be drawn in by the snazzy tagline, or the 'nutritious' revamped formula – the newly responsible 'holistic approach'. None of these things matter – they're just distractions from the core message and ideology. The only way to be healthy (and to maintain a healthy weight, if that's your concern) is to have a balanced, nutritious lifestyle which incorporates exercise and isn't temporary or geared towards 'weight loss'.

3/ *Healthy eating should be for life* – *and it shouldn't be complicated or miserable*

Part of the reason diets are unhealthy (and don't work) is that they offer a temporary 'solution' – a sticking plaster. They don't offer you sustained good health or benefit your body in any way. The only way to do this is to start to think of food and your body in a different light, and live your life in a way that makes you healthy and happy. This involves not focusing on weight or calories. Instead it involves changing your perspective on fat and nutrition altogether. Most importantly, it involves giving your body the best you possibly can and not abusing it in any way – in the long-term, not just for a few weeks.

10. Further reading and extra resources

I learnt a lot about nutrition from reputable sites and studies I found online, but with so many irresponsible sources of information I thought it would be handy to include some of the sites I find useful myself here in the book.

www.authoritynutrition.com

www.mercola.com

www.whfoods.com

Other books by Rose

TOUGH COOKIE

ANOREXIA: THE BARE BONES

EATING DISORDERS: PARENT HANDBOOK

TOUGH LOVE

RECIPES FOR RECOVERY series

RECIPES FOR RECOVERY: THE SWEET STUFF series

Visit www.toughcookieblog.co.uk to purchase and find out more, or search for me on Amazon and Barnes and Noble: **Rose Walters Tough Cookie** and follow the links to my Author Page.

www.ingramcontent.com/pod-product-compliance
Lightning Source LLC
Chambersburg PA
CBHW060426290526
45791CB00002B/882